Eat to Live Diet Reloaded:

70 Top Eat to Live Recipes You Will Love!

Table of Contents

Advantages of Going on a Nutrient Rich Diet

Using natural and organic food as a way to improve one's well-being is not a new concept at all.

Ancient people from past civilizations thrived well on a diet of organic and natural grown food. They also learned how to utilize particular plants for medicinal purposes.

Unfortunately, with the emergence of the Industrial period, and the introduction of sugar into our diets, many of us have fallen into the trap of eating "convenient" food items (a.k.a. processed food,) and drinks that have extremely high levels of sugar. Time and time again, these have proven to be detrimental to our health.

Going back to the basics and subscribing to a nutrient rich diet, you can:

1. <u>Lose weight naturally, gradually and safely</u>. Because this diet is high in essential nutrients and low in fat, sugar, and salt, it is relatively easier to shed off the unwanted poundage by simply adhering to the principles of the diet. More importantly, you do no put yourself at risk (or complicate existing health issues, if any) by following a diet that encourages rapid weight loss in a short amount of time.

Although this may sound counterintuitive, gradually losing weight over a longer period is actually a far better option than dropping excess pounds in just a few weeks or days. For starters, crash dieting would only compromise the health of your internal organs: your liver and kidneys, in particular. This could lead to lifelong and potentially dangerous health complications like: all manner of liver diseases and kidney failure.

Secondly, crash dieting is often interpreted by the body as a period of starvation: a state wherein your internal organs experience extreme nutrient deprivation. Because there is no longer an external source of nutrients, the body turns inward. It burns off its store of reserved fat in the adipose tissues. In extreme cases, the body can even burn off muscle cells to acquire a protein source. This is the real reason why people lose weight when they crash diet.

Unfortunately, once the diet is over, the body autonomically (without conscious thought on your part) takes extreme measures to ensure that it does not undergo starvation again. The first thing it does is to create voluminous amount of adipose tissues around the abdominal area, the thighs and the butt. Any fat or oil you eat afterwards are deposited into these tissues, and are reserved for later use.

This makes it easy to rapidly regain all the weight you've lost before, and then some! Worse, because the body is "reserving" the stored fat, it becomes harder to lose the excess pounds afterwards.

With a nutrient rich diet though, your weight loss is safer and definitely more sustainable in the long run.

2.   Helps stabilize your blood sugar. This is especially beneficial to diabetics or those who are already in the pre-diabetic stage. A nutrient rich diet discourages the excessive consumption of table sugar or other sweeteners that can alter the balance of insulin in the bloodstream.

An imbalance of insulin can lead to other health issues like: hyperglycemia (high levels of blood sugar due to low insulin in the bloodstream,) hypoglycemia (low levels of blood sugar due to excessive insulin intake or production,) blindness, obesity, and kidney failure, etc. It can also complicate existing heart, liver, and kidney conditions.

For people with Type I diabetes, uncontrolled hyperglycemia increases the risk of diabetic coma; while uncontrolled hypoglycemia can lead to insulin shock that could lead to diabetic coma as well. This is a life-threatening condition that would need medical intervention.

3.   Helps stabilize your blood's cholesterol level. A diet high in oils and fats can dramatically increase your cholesterol level. This can cause: liver and kidney failure, obesity, diabetes, etc. Unfortunately, having high cholesterol also causes 2 life-threatening conditions, namely: heart failure (congestive cardiac failure) and stroke (cerebrovascular accident.)

With a nutrient rich diet though, the intake of oils and fats are limited. This lowers *all* the risks normally associated with high blood pressure due to unhealthy blood cholesterol level.

At the same, this diet does not completely removed oils and fats from its prescribed meals, as these are also nutrients essential to keep hair, nails and skin healthy. The key is to find healthier options or alternatives, and to keep portions small.

* ~ *

Rediscovering the taste and benefits of naturally grown and organic food can improve your health greatly. These recipes are incredibly easy to make too. Aside from helping you save a lot of money, these recipes are proven to yield tasty and delicious food and beverages each and every time.

So if you are ready, here are 70 recipes you might want to incorporate in your daily meals.

Salad Recipes

Fresh, crisp, green salads *should* constitute the majority of your meals. These are incredibly healthy, tasty, and have very few calories. This is why you can consume as much of these as you want. You can even use these as side dishes for meals, or slide these in with your favorite sandwiches and burgers for a heftier snack.

In order to keep things healthy though, here are a few ground rules:

1.   <u>Fresh vegetables are always the best</u>. Although you can use frozen or canned food items like carrots, corn, green peas, etc. as substitutes for fresh produce, you have to remember that some of the essential nutrients may have been lost through the processing stage. Limit the use of frozen or canned food items as much as possible.

If you have to use these, thaw frozen vegetables completely in the fridge to preserve its flavor. If using canned vegetables, wash these thoroughly under cool, running water to remove excess starch, salt and sugar.

2.   <u>Raw and fresh fruits are better than canned and bottled ones</u>. Raw and fresh fruits provide 100% more nutrients than their processed counterparts. These also contain less sugar.

If you would like to incorporate fruit juice into your salads, always use freshly squeezed ones. And squeeze these just before you are about to serve or eat the salad. Use fruit pulp and zest whenever possible.

3.   <u>Be adventurous when it comes to trying out new fruits and vegetables</u>. If you limit yourself to the few produce you know, chances are: you will end up with a boring diet. There are numerous fruits and vegetables you can try that will help you eat healthier and even offer you new dishes to love. So be brave when it comes to eating healthier.

4.   <u>Keep your salad dressings simple and separate</u>. Your healthy salads could quickly turn into an unhealthy bowl of processed food if you keep using ready made condiments, dips and dressings. To adhere to the principles of this diet, you need to learn how to make your own dips and dressings from scratch.

This is the only way to ascertain exactly what goes into your own food. You can also find healthier alternatives to sugar, and control the amount of salt or oil when you make your own meals.

Note: recipes for dips and dressings are on Chapter 3.

Broccoli and Cauliflower Salad

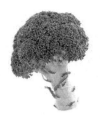

Ingredients:

2	heads	broccoli, washed, drained, cut into bite-sized florets
1	head	cauliflower, washed, drained, cut into bite-sized florets
-	dash	garlic powder
-	dash	olive oil
-	-	salt to taste
-	-	white pepper to taste (optional)
-	-	water

You would also need: ice bath (a bowl of water and ice cubes)
strainer or colander
slotted spoon

Directions:

1.   Halfway fill a deep saucepan with water. Allow water to boil over medium heat.

2.   Gently slide in the broccoli and cauliflower florets into the boiling liquid. Turn the heat off and put the lid on. Allow the vegetables to sit in the cooking water for only a minute.

3.   With a slotted spoon, remove vegetables immediately out of the water and into the ice bath. This stops the cooking process and would help keep the broccoli and cauliflower crisp and vibrant looking. Drain vegetables into a strainer after 2 minutes.

4.   Transfer the broccoli and cauliflower florets into another bowl and season with the remaining ingredients. Serve immediately.

Cold White Bean Salad

Ingredients:

For the stew:

2	cups	dried small white beans, washed and drained well (You can substitute dried *cannellini* or navy beans.)
6	cups	water
1	cup	black or green olives in brine, washed thoroughly under running water, drained well, pitted then halved
-	-	salt to taste
-	-	black pepper to taste

For the emulsion:

¼	cup	white wine or apple cider vinegar
½	cup	extra virgin olive oil
2	tbsp.	Dijon or yellow mustard
2	pieces	garlic cloves, peeled and grated

For the salad:

1	head	lettuce of your choice, leaves washed individually, drained well, leaves torn into bite size pieces
2	pieces	tomatoes, medium-sized, washed, and cut into wedges

You would also need: slow cooker
strainer or colander
wire whisk

Directions:

1.   Set the slow cooker at its lowest setting. Place the beans and water in. Cook for 8 hours, or until beans are soft enough to be mashed between your fingers. Carefully pour the beans into a strainer. Wash beans under running water. Drain well before transferring to a large glass bowl.

2.   In a separate bowl, combine all the ingredients of the emulsion. Whisk vigorously until liquid turns cloudy. Pour this over the beans and toss gently. Add the

green onions and olives. Season to taste with salt and pepper. Chill for at least an hour before serving.

3.   To assemble: line a plate with torn lettuce leaves and a few pieces of tomato wedges. Ladle a generous serving of the chilled white beans on top. Serve with bread or soup.

Green Beans and Asparagus Salad

Ingredients:

½	pound	fresh snap beans, washed, ends and strings removed (You can substitute *edamame,* Romano or French green beans.)
½	pound	white asparagus, choose the ones with thicker stems, washed, tough ends snapped off and sliced roughly the same length of the snap beans
5	pieces	garlic cloves, peeled and minced
1	tbsp.	olive oil
-	-	water
-	-	salt to taste
-	-	pepper to taste

You would also need: strainer or colander
                          slotted spoon

Directions:

1.   In a skillet, heat the oil until slightly smoky. Quickly sauté the minced garlic until it turns lightly brown and aromatic. Remove skillet from flame and allow to cool at room temperature. Keep a careful eye on the garlic as this could still burn. If the garlic seems to be getting browner, simply remove the garlic pieces with a slotted spoon and set aside.

2.   In a deep stock pot, add the string beans and cover with water. Bring to a gentle boil, about 3 minutes. Quickly toss in the asparagus slivers and allow to cook for about 1 minute more. Quickly but carefully drain the vegetables into the strainer.

3.   Toss drained vegetables into the garlic oil and coat the vegetables well. If you have separated the minced garlic from the oil, simply toss the toasted garlic on top of the coated vegetables. Season with salt and pepper. Serve immediately.

Mushroom Salad in *Teriyaki* Sauce

Ingredients:

1	tbsp.	extra virgin olive oil
½	pound	canned button mushrooms, washed under running water, drained well, sliced into thin slivers
¼	cup	*teriyaki* sauce

For the salad:

3	handfuls	salad greens of your choice, washed, drained and torn into bite size pieces, chilled
1	cup	grape tomatoes, washed, stems removed, halved, chilled
1	piece	cucumber, washed, ends removed, cubed, chilled
1	stalk	celery, washed, roots trimmed, coarsely chopped, chilled

For the garnish:

1	stalk	scallion, washed, roots trimmed, coarsely chopped
1	tsp.	sesame seeds, toasted on a dry frying pan, cooled to room temperature

Directions:

1.   Place the oil on the skillet and turn the heat up on its highest setting. Caramelize the mushroom slices for about 2 minutes. Turn the heat down.

2.   Carefully pour the *teriyaki* sauce into the hot skillet and allow this to simmer for a few seconds. Remove from flame and allow to cool completely. Chill the sauce for an hour, if possible.

3.   Toss all the salad ingredients well into a large glass bowl. Toss with the mushrooms and the *teriyaki* sauce. Garnish with scallions and sesame seeds just before serving.

Warm Broccoli and Mushroom Salad

Ingredients:

1	head	fresh broccoli, large-sized, washed, dried and cut into bite-sized florets
1	tsp.	extra virgin olive oil
¼	cup	onion, peeled and finely diced
2	tbsp.	balsamic vinegar
3	cups	canned button mushrooms, washed under running water, drained well, quartered
-	-	water
-	-	salt

You would also need: slotted spoon
ice bath (bowl of water and ice)

Directions:

1.   Halfway fill a small saucepan with water. Add a pinch of salt and set it over high flame. Wait for the water to boil before sliding in the broccoli florets. Cover saucepan. After 2 minutes, remove the vegetables from the hot water with a slotted spoon. Place broccoli immediately into the ice bath to stop the cooking process. Set aside.

2.   In a skillet, heat the oil until slightly smoky. Stir fry the onions until wilted, about 1 minute. Carefully pour in the balsamic vinegar. Let this cook until the liquid is reduced in half. This should take no more than 30 seconds. Remove skillet from flame.

3. To assemble: in a serving or casserole dish, toss the mushrooms and the drained broccoli florets together. Season with more salt, if needed. Serve immediately.

Condiments, Dips and Dressing Recipes

Avocado and Tomato Dip

Ingredients:

4	cups	fresh, ripe cherry tomatoes, washed, halved
1	piece	very ripe avocado, medium-sized, stone removed, flesh scooped out
2	tbsp.	freshly squeezed lemon or lime juice, include as much of the pulp as possible, seeds removed
1	handful	fresh cilantro or parsley, washed and dried
-	-	salt to taste
-	-	pepper to taste

You would also need: food processor or blender

Directions:

Process all the ingredients together, except the salt and pepper. Pulse 5 to 7 times for a chunky consistency. Process for 20 seconds or more for a smoother dip. Chill before serving.

Avocado and Grapefruit Chunky Dip

Ingredients:

1	piece	overripe avocado, medium-sized, stone removed, flesh scooped out, then mashed roughly with a fork
1	piece	grapefruit, peeled, membranes and seeds removed, shred the pulp using your fingers, reserve any grapefruit juice
1	piece	Japanese cucumber, medium-sized, washed, dried, ends and seeds removed, minced
2	pieces	celery stalks, leaves removed, roots trimmed, minced
-	-	salt to taste
-	-	pepper to taste

Directions:

Combine everything in a bowl and season well. Chill before serving. This is perfect for toasted pita bread or vegetable sticks.

Babaganouj

ngredients:

2	pieces	large eggplants, washed and dried, stems trimmed
½	cup	*tahini*
¼	tsp.	cumin powder
1	piece	garlic clove, peeled
1	dash	garlic powder
1	dash	onion powder
-	-	olive oil or any vegetable oil

You will also need:
- oven
- baking dish
- food processor or blender
- spoon
- fork

Directions:

1. Preheat oven to 400°F or 200°C.

2. Lightly brush baking dish with olive oil. Place eggplants whole on the baking surface and bake for 30 to 45 minutes. The flesh of the eggplant should be completely soft. Test by pricking with a fork.

3. Remove eggplants from oven and allow to cool completely at room temperature. Once cooled, cut the eggplants lengthwise. Using a spoon, carefully scrape off the seed row and discard. Scrape the remaining flesh into the food processor, along with the remaining ingredients.

4. Process to desired consistency. Some people like this chunky, while others prefer a smoother dip. If you like the chunkier version, process only for a few seconds. A longer processing time will create a thicker but smoother paste. Serve warm.

Berry and *Tahini* Dip

Ingredients:

4	cups	cherry tomatoes, washed and halved
1	cup	fresh or frozen blueberries (You can substitute fresh or frozen strawberries, or any berries that are in season.)
3	tbsp.	*tahini* or almond butter
1	tbsp.	freshly squeezed lemon or lime juice
1	handful	fresh cilantro or parsley, coarsely chopped
-	-	salt to taste
-	-	pepper to taste

You would also need: food processor or blender

Directions:

Except for the salt and pepper, process everything until you have a smooth consistency. Chill for at least 15 minutes before using. Season to taste. Add more lemon juice if desired.

Blueberry Dip

Ingredients:

1½	cups	fresh or frozen blueberries, washed and drained well
2	pieces	fresh dates, pitted, washed and drained well
1	tbsp.	apple cider vinegar
1	tbsp.	freshly squeezed lemon, use as much of the pulp as possible
-	-	salt to taste
-	-	pepper to taste

You would also need: food processor or blender

Directions:

Process all the ingredients, except for the salt and pepper. Transfer to a glass container and chill for at least 15 minutes. Season well with salt and pepper just before serving.

Dill and Tomato Dip

Ingredients:

2	pieces	ripe tomatoes, washed and halved
1	tsp.	*tahini* or almond butter
2	tsp.	freshly squeezed lemon juice
-	dash	fresh or dried dill
-	-	salt to taste
-	-	pepper to taste

You would also need: food processor or blender

Directions:

Process everything except the salt and pepper. Add more dill or *tahini*, desired. Season well with salt and pepper. Chill before serving.

Garlic and Ginger Salad Dressing

Ingredients:

1	knob	fresh ginger root, thumb-sized, washed, peeled and grated, stringy parts discarded
2	pieces	garlic cloves, peeled and grated
4	tbsp.	light soy sauce
4	tbsp.	water
4	tsp.	freshly squeezed lemon juice
2	tsp.	apple cider vinegar

You would also need: grater

Directions:

In a bowl, mix all the ingredients together. Pour over salad greens only before serving.

Herb Dip with Sun Dried Tomatoes

Ingredients:

1	cup	fresh mint leaves, lightly packed, washed, stems removed
½	cup	fresh cilantro leaves, lightly packed, washed
¼	cup	fresh chives, lightly packed, washed, roots removed, choose only the green part of the leaves
4	pieces	sun dried tomatoes, coarsely chopped
3	tbsp.	water
2	tbsp.	freshly squeezed lemon juice
-	-	salt to taste
-	-	pepper to taste

You would also need: food processor or blender

Directions:

Place the mint leaves, cilantro, chives and tomatoes into the food processor. Add the lemon juice and blend until you have a smooth consistency. If the dip is too thick, add water 1 tablespoon at a time. Season well with salt and pepper. Serve immediately.

Hot Pepper Dressing

Ingredients:

1	piece	fresh *jalapeño* pepper or bird's eye pepper, washed, stalk removed (If you prefer a milder taste, carefully remove the seeds of the pepper. If not, leave the pepper intact.)
1	piece	garlic clove, peeled, halved
1	piece	onion, small-sized, peeled, sliced into wedges
1	knob	fresh ginger, thumb-sized, washed, peeled
1	cup	water
-	-	salt to taste
-	-	pepper to taste

You will also need: food processor or blender

Directions:

Place everything in the food processor and blend well. You can use this as salad dressing or sauce for meals. Adjust seasoning according to taste.

Mango Dip

Ingredients:

4	pieces	tomatoes, large-sized, washed, dried, coarsely chopped
2	pieces	ripe mangoes, medium-sized, stones removed, flesh scooped out
4	tbsp.	apple cider vinegar
½	cup	water
-	-	salt to taste
-	-	white pepper to taste

You would also need: food processor or blender

Directions:

Except for the salt and white pepper, simply process all the ingredients together until you have a smooth consistency. Season according to taste and chill before serving.

Legume and Grain Based Meals

Bean and Corn Salad

Ingredients:

1	cup	boiled kidney beans (You can substitute canned beans but wash these first to remove excess salt and sugar,) drained
1	cup	boiled pinto beans (You can substitute canned beans but wash these first to remove excess salt and sugar,) drained
1	cup	boiled corn kernels (You can substitute canned or frozen whole corn kernels but wash these first to remove excess salt and sugar,) drained
1	piece	yellow bell pepper, washed, cored, seeds removed, diced
1	piece	red bell pepper, washed, cored, seeds removed, diced
2	pieces	garlic cloves, peeled, crushed (for a milder taste,) or minced (for a sharper taste)
1	handful	fresh cilantro leaves, washed, coarsely chopped
1	piece	lemon, medium-sized, halved, seeded and juiced
1	tsp.	cumin powder (You can substitute all spice powder.)
¼	cup	soy oil
-	-	salt to taste
-	-	pepper to taste
1	piece	jalapeño pepper, diced (optional)

Directions:

Toss all the ingredients together in a large bowl. Make sure that you coat everything well with the soy oil. Adjust the taste by adding more salt and pepper, if needed. Use the jalapeño pepper if you want a spicier salad. Chill for an hour before serving.

Beans and Peas Salad

Ingredients:

1	pound	frozen green peas, completely thawed in the fridge, drained
1	pound	chickpeas, cooked, drained (You can substitute canned chickpeas.)
1	pound	kidney beans, cooked, drained (You can substitute canned kidney beans.)
5	pieces	garlic cloves, peeled and minced

For the vinaigrette:

3	tbsp.	extra virgin olive oil
3	tbsp.	apple cider vinegar
-	-	salt to taste
-	-	pepper to taste

Directions:

In a large skillet, heat the oil up until slightly smoky. Add the minced garlic until it is lightly brown and aromatic. Remove quickly from the fire. Toss in the green peas, chickpeas, and kidney beans. Mix well. Season to taste, and serve immediately.

Carrot with Cashew in Rice Stew

Ingredients:

2	tbsp.	extra virgin olive oil
3	pieces	onions, medium-sized, peeled and minced
½	head	cabbage, medium-sized, washed, julienned, drained well
1	piece	carrot, medium-sized, peeled and minced
1	piece	apple, large-sized, washed, peeled, cored and minced
½	cup	raisins
½	cup	whole raw cashew nuts
8	cups	vegetable stock
¼	cup	tomato paste
½	cup	brown, red or wild rice, washed under running water until the liquid turns clear, drained well
-	-	salt and pepper taste
-	-	water as needed

Directions:

1.   In a Dutch oven, heat the oil over medium flame. Sauté the onion until it turns transparent. Add in the cabbage and carrots. Stir fry for a minute or until shredded cabbage turns limp.

2.   Carefully pour the vegetable stock and the tomato paste into the Dutch oven. Turn the flame up to its highest setting and bring the stew to a boil.

3.   Add in the washed rice, cashew nuts and the apple slices. Reduce heat to the lowest setting and stir to prevent the rice from sticking to the bottom of the pot. Place the lid on and allow this to simmer until the rice is cooked through. This should take between 20 to 35 minutes.

After 20 minutes, check the rice if it can easily be mashed by a fork. Continue with the next step if the rice is soft enough. If not, continue cooking for another 5 minutes. There should still be a lot of liquid in the pot. However, if the rice has absorbed most of the liquid, add water one cup at a time to prevent the stew from drying out.

4.   Stir in the raisins. Season with salt and pepper. Remove stew from flame. Serve warm.

Couscous and Vegetable Salad

Ingredients:

1	cup	couscous, choose the easy-to-cook or instant variety
1	cup	boiling water
1	head	cauliflower, washed, dried and cut into florets
1	piece	carrot, medium-sized, washed, peeled, diced
1	piece	green bell pepper, small-sized, washed, seeded, diced
1	piece	shallot, peeled, minced
$\frac{1}{3}$	cup	canned chickpeas, wash under running water, drained well
½	cup	sun dried tomatoes
¼	cup	black olives in brine, coarsely chopped
½	tsp.	allspice powder
½	tsp.	cumin powder
-	-	zest of 2 lemons
2	pieces	lemons, halved and squeezed, seeds removed
¼	cup	extra virgin olive oil
-	-	salt to taste

You would also need: saran wrap
ice bath (bowl of water and ice)
strainer or colander
slotted spoon

Directions:

1.   In a large heat-resistant bowl, combine boiling water and couscous together. Stir once, then cover the bowl with saran wrap. Set aside for 5 minutes to let the couscous absorb the liquid. After 5 minutes, remove the cover and fluff the couscous by gently working it with a fork. Cover with saran wrap again and set aside.

2.   In a small pot, place the sun dried tomatoes and cover with an inch of water. Allow the water to simmer gently for 5 minutes. Fish the tomatoes out of the pot and chop these into large chunks. Set aside to cool.

3.   Meanwhile, halfway fill a separate pot with water. Allow water to boil before carefully sliding in the diced carrots and cauliflower florets. Cook for 5 minutes. With a slotted spoon, remove the vegetables from the pot and place it into the ice bath.

4.   Place the couscous in a tight mesh strainer. Wash under running water to remove excess starch. Drain the couscous well before using.

5.   In a large bowl, toss all the vegetables and spices together, including the lemon juice, lemon zest, and extra virgin olive oil. Season well with salt. Add the couscous and mix gently but thoroughly. Refrigerate until you are ready to serve.

De-constructed Cheese-less, Nut-Free Pesto Pasta

1	pound	spinach and/or carrot flavored *fettuccine*, cooked according to package instructions, drained well. Drizzle oil to prevent the strands from sticking together. Set aside. (You can substitute any regular ribbon pasta, such as: *linguine, pappardelle, tagliatelle,* or spaghetti.)
1	handful	fresh basil leaves, washed, stems removed, coarsely chopped
2	pieces	fresh tomatoes, large-sized, halved, seeds removed, julienned
5	pieces	garlic cloves, peeled and grated
2	tbsp.	balsamic vinegar
¼	cup	extra virgin olive oil
-	-	salt to taste
-	-	pepper to taste

You would also need: whisk

Directions:

1.   Combine oil with balsamic vinegar and minced garlic. Whisk well until it emulsifies a little. Add the chopped basil leaves. Season with salt and pepper.

2.   Pour this emulsion into the cooked pasta and toss gently but thoroughly. Make sure that each strand of the pasta is well coated with the flavored oil.

3.   Just before serving, add the tomato slices and toss again. Serve immediately.

Fusilli in Garden Salad with Apple Cider Vinaigrette

Ingredients:

2	cups	spinach and/or carrot *fusilli* or corkscrew pasta, cooked according to package directions, drizzled with a little olive oil to prevent pasta strands from sticking together. Chill in the fridge as soon as possible. (You can substitute plain *fusilli*, or other cut pasta like: *cavatappi, gemelli, penne,* or *ziti.*)
1	head	broccoli, washed and cut into florets
1	piece	large carrot, washed, peeled, sliced roughly into the size of the cooked pasta, chilled
1	piece	large cucumber, washed, ends removed, skin left intact, sliced roughly the size of the cooked pasta, chilled
1	piece	large tomato, washed, sliced in half to remove seeds, sliced roughly the size of the cooked pasta, chilled
-	-	water

For the vinaigrette:

2	tbsp.	olive oil
2	tbsp.	apple cider vinegar
1	tsp.	dried basil
-	-	salt to taste
-	-	white pepper to taste

You would also need: ice bath (a bowl of water and ice cubes)
wire whisk
slotted spoon

Directions:
1.   Halfway fill a small saucepan with water. Bring to boil. Gently slide in the broccoli florets and carrot slices. Cook covered for 1 minute. Turn heat off. With a slotted spoon, scoop vegetables into the ice bath to stop the cooking process. Set aside.

2.   In a bowl, whisk together all the ingredients for the vinaigrette until mixture emulsifies slightly. Season to taste.

3.   Just before serving, remove the broccoli and carrots from the ice bath and drain well. In another bowl, combine the cooked pasta and all the vegetables. Drizzle the vinaigrette over the pasta and toss. Serve immediately.

Harira (Lentil and Bean Soup)

Ingredients:

1	tbsp.	extra virgin olive oil
2	pieces	onions, medium-sized, peeled and minced
2	tsp.	curry powder
1	tsp.	ground cumin powder
2	tsp.	fresh rosemary leaves, washed, needles coarsely chopped (You can substitute 1 tsp. dried rosemary leaves or dried rosemary powder.)
1	tsp.	fennel seeds
6	cups	vegetable stock
1	cup	dried white beans
1	cup	dried red lentils
½	cup	red or brown or wild rice
1	piece	tomato, medium-sized, sliced in half to remove seeds, diced
½	cup	fresh cilantro leaves, reserve a few sprigs for garnish later, washed, stems removed, coarsely chopped
1	tbsp.	tomato paste
-	-	salt to taste
-	-	black pepper to taste
-	-	Tabasco sauce to taste
-	-	water as needed

Directions:

1.   Heat oil in a Dutch oven. Cook onions until transparent. This would take no more than 5 minutes. Add the herbs and spices: cumin, curry powder, fennel seeds and chopped rosemary leaves.

2.   Pour in the vegetable stock, along with the beans, lentils and rice. Turn the heat on its highest setting and bring the stew to a boil, uncovered. Stir frequently to ensure that the rice and legumes do not stick to the bottom of the Dutch oven.

3.   Once the stew comes to comes to a boil, turn the the heat down to the lowest setting, and allow stew to simmer gently for the next 30 minutes, partly covered. After 30 minutes, test rice, beans and lentils if these are cooked through and can be mashed by a fork. If not, add more water, one cup at a time to keep the stew from drying out.

4.   If the rice and legumes are cooked, add in the diced tomatoes and tomato paste. These only have to be heated through. Season well with salt, pepper and Tabasco sauce. Remove from flame. Garnish with cilantro sprigs just before serving.

Lo Mein, Mushroom and Vegetable Salad

Ingredients:

1	pound	dried *lo mein* noodles, cooked according to package directions then set aside to cool completely at room temperature (You can substitute *soba* noodles or any dried, round egg noodles. Spaghetti also works fine in a pinch.)
3	tbsp.	roasted sesame oil
1	head	broccoli, medium-sized, washed, dried and cut into florets
4	pieces	*bok choy* leaves, washed, roots trimmed, sliced diagonally into ½ inch slivers
1	piece	carrot, large-sized, washed, peeled and julienned
1	piece	red bell pepper, medium-sized, washed, cored, seeded and julienned
4	large	fresh *portobello* mushrooms, stalks removed, caps sliced thinly (You can substitute fresh button mushrooms. Canned *portobello* and button mushrooms can be used in a pinch. Wash these thoroughly under running water and drain well before using.)
¼	cup	water
2	tbsp.	light soy sauce
2	tbsp.	apple cider vinegar
3	tbsp.	sesame seeds, freshly toasted on a frying pan just before using

You would also need: strainer or colander

Directions:

1.   Drizzle sesame oil on the cooked noodles. With clean hands, gently massage the oil into the cooked noodles to loosen strands up. Set aside.

2.   Fill a saucepan halfway with water. Bring to boil. Turn heat down, then add all the vegetables all at once: broccoli, *bok choy* leaves, carrots and the sliced *portobello* mushrooms. Boil for only 2 minutes.

3.   Drain the vegetables using the strainer. Discard the cooking liquid. Gently let running water wash over the cooked vegetables to ensure that these remain crisp when you eat them. Drain well.

4.   In a large glass bowl, combine the the noodles, cooked vegetables and the remaining ingredients and toss lightly. Chill before serving.

Tabouli

Ingredients:

½	cup	*bulgar* wheat (choose the easy-to-cook or instant variety)
1	cup	water
1	piece	shallot, small-sized, peeled, washed and diced
1	piece	green bell pepper, washed, stem removed, cored, seeded and diced
1	piece	tomato, large-sized, halved to remove seeds, diced
1	handful	flat leaf parsley, washed, stems removed, chopped roughly
1	piece	lemon, juiced, seeds removed
2	tbsp.	extra virgin olive oil
-	-	salt to taste

Directions:

1.   In a saucepan, combine the *bulgar* wheat and the water. Mix well then bring to a boil. Reduce the heat after 3 minutes. Remove the saucepan from the fire then cover with a lid. Let this stand undisturbed for the next 20 to 30 minutes. Remove the lid afterwards to speed up the cooling process. Once the saucepan is cool enough to touch, transfer this to the fridge to cool further.

2.	Meanwhile, combine the rest of the ingredients in a large glass bowl. Mix well and season with salt. Chill this mixture in the fridge until the bulgar is ready.

3.	To serve, toss the chilled *bulgar* with the mixed vegetables. Serve as a side dish or as a meal in itself.

Wari Muth (Black Beans with Garan Masala)

Ingredients:

2	cups	dried black beans, washed, dried
6	cups	water
½	tsp.	dried red pepper flakes
2	tsp.	fennel seeds, roughly pounded into a coarse paste
1	tsp.	*garan masala* (You can substitute curry powder.)
1	tsp.	ground ginger powder
2	tsp.	turmeric powder
-	-	salt to taste
¼	cup	fresh cilantro leaves, coarsely chopped for garnish

You would also need:	slow cooker

Directions:

Except for the salt and the garnish, place everything in the slow cooker and stir once. Place a lid on and set the cooker on the highest setting. After an hour, turn the cooker down to its lowest setting. Allow beans to cook undisturbed for the next 7 hours. Season well with salt just before serving. Top with chopped cilantro leaves.

Homemade Breads

When creating breads from scratch, it is essential to learn at least one basic recipe. This will make it easier to create more complicated breads in the future.

Basic Artisan Bread Recipe (BABR)

With this recipe, you do not need to:

* Proof yeast,
* Knead the dough,
* Punch down the dough and let it rise again,
* Worry that dough did not rise high or long enough,
* Worry that dough will fall flat after a long rising period, and
* Make a new batch of dough every time you need bread.

Ingredients:

5½	cups	whole wheat flour
2¼	cups	all purpose flour (plus a few more for dusting later)
1½	tsp. / 0.55 oz.	granulated or fast acting yeast
1	tbsp.	rock or kosher salt
4	cups	lukewarm water
2	cups	cornmeal for dusting (plus a few more for dusting later)
-	dash	whole seed mixtures for topping, like: raw caraway seeds, flaxseed, raw sunflower seeds, poppy and sesame seeds

You would also need:
large mixing bowls
saran wrap
oven
baking sheets or silicone mat
parchment paper
pizza peel or upside down baking sheet
kitchen shears
baking stone or thick-bottomed baking sheet
metal broiler tray
pastry brush

sharp knife
wire rack
wire whisk
wooden spoon (optional)

Directions:

1.   In a large bowl, whisk together the 2 flours, yeast and salt.

2.   Make sure that the water is still slightly warmer than body temperature before adding this to the dry ingredients.

3.   Mix flour and water using a wooden spoon, or preferably with your clean, bare hands. Make sure that everything is evenly incorporated and that there are no longer any patches of dry flour.

4.   Cover the bowl loosely with saran wrap. Let the dough rise. Set this in a warm, dry place where it can remain undisturbed for at least 2 hours. However, the longer this dough remains undisturbed, the better its flavor becomes.

5.   After the preferred rising period, transfer the loosely covered bowl into the fridge. The dough will retain its "freshness" for the next 14 days. This step also makes the dough easier to work with. Whatever you do, do not punch down the dough, or you will end up with an incredibly dense bread.

6.   If you are ready to bake, prepare your pizza peel by dusting it generously with cornmeal. If you are using a baking sheet, turn this upside down and line the bottom with silicone mat or with parchment paper. Dust the surface with cornmeal.

7.   Retrieve the chilled dough from the fridge. Remove the cover and lightly dust the surface of the dough with all purpose flour.

8.   Pull up a grapefruit size (approximately 1 pound) dough, and cut it off using your kitchen shears. Add a little more flour to both your hands and the dough so that you can shape it into a ball.

9.   Gently tug on the surface of the dough and tuck it underneath. This will help create the crust of the bread. Repeat this step as often as needed to form a smooth surface. This process should be done quickly. About 20 to 40 seconds is enough. Otherwise, all the air inside the dough would escape, and the bread will become dense and chewy after baking.

10.   Now shape the dough into a loaf, and place it bottom side down on the pizza peel. Let this rest for another 90 minutes. Cover dough loaf loosely with saran wrap. If the saran wrap seems to be sticking to the surface of the dough, dust again with a light layer of flour.

At this stage, the dough will look like it is deflating. Do not panic. The bread will start to rise once it gets into the hot oven.

11.   30 minutes before baking, heat the oven up to 400°F or 200°C. Place the baking stone on the middle rack of the oven. If you don't have a baking stone, just use a thick-bottomed baking sheet large enough to accommodate the size of your dough loaf.

12.   Place an empty metal broiler tray on the rack underneath the baking stone.

13.   Just before baking, diagonally score the surface of the dough with a sharp knife. Two ¼ inch deep slashes would suffice.

14.   Using a pastry brush dipped in a small amount of water, gently brush off the excess flour on the surface of the dough.

15.   Lightly sprinkle your preferred whole seed mixture topping.

16.   Prepare 1 cup of hot water before you open the oven door.

17.   Very carefully but quickly transfer the dough from the pizza peel and unto the hot baking stone. If you have to gently move the dough with your hand, do so but be careful of the hot surfaces. If you are using parchment paper or silicone mat, simply tug the paper or mat unto the baking stone.

18.   Pour the cup of hot water into the empty metal broiler tray underneath the baking stone.

19.   Quickly close the oven door to trap in the steam and continue baking the bread at this temperature for 30 to 40 minutes. The bread is done when the crust turns golden brown.

20.   Remove the bread from the oven. Allow this to cool completely on a wire rack before slicing or serving it. This will help create a crisp crust but soft interior. Cooling time may take between 15 to 45 minutes, depending on room temperature.

Basil and Pine Nut Loaf

This recipe follows the Basic Artisan Bread Recipe (BABR) on page 32, but includes these...

Ingredients:

2	tsp.	fresh basil leaves, washed, dried, stems removed, and leaves coarsely chopped (You can substitute 1 tsp. of dried basil. Do not use dried basil powder.)
4	tsp.	raw pine nuts, coarsely crushed

From the BABR recipe, you need to remove this:

dash	whole seed mixtures for topping, like: raw caraway seeds, flaxseed, raw sunflower seeds, poppy and sesame seeds

Directions:

1.   Follow BABR directions. But in step 2, incorporate basil leaves and crushed pine nuts with the lukewarm water.

2.   Proceed with the steps 3 to 14.

3.   Skip step 15, then proceed with the remaining steps.

Black and Green Olive Loaf

This recipe follows the Basic Artisan Bread Recipe (BABR) on page 32, but includes these...

Ingredients:

| 4 | pieces | black olives in brine or oil, washed thoroughly, dried, pits removed and minced (Do not use fresh olives as these become bitter during the long rising process.) |
| 4 | pieces | green olives in brine or oil, washed thoroughly, dried, pits removed and minced (Do not use fresh olives as these become bitter during the long rising process.) |

From the BABR recipe, you need to remove this:

| | dash | whole seed mixtures for topping, like: raw caraway seeds, flaxseed, raw sunflower seeds, poppy and sesame seeds |

Directions:

1.   Follow BABR directions. But in step 2, incorporate the olives with the lukewarm water.

2.   Proceed with the steps 3 to 14.

3.   Skip step 15, then proceed with the remaining steps.

Easy Onion Sourdough Loaf

This recipe follows the Basic Artisan Bread Recipe (BABR) on page 32, but includes these...

Ingredients:

4	tsp.	fresh leeks, choose only the green parts, washed and minced
1	tbsp	white wine vinegar

From the BABR recipe, you need to remove this:

dash	whole seed mixtures for topping, like: raw caraway seeds, flaxseed, raw sunflower seeds, poppy and sesame seeds

Directions:

1.   Follow BABR directions. But in step 2, incorporate the leeks and the white wine vinegar with the lukewarm water.

2.   Proceed with the steps 3 to 14.

3.   Skip step 15, then proceed with the remaining steps.

Garlic and Parsley Loaf

This recipe follows the Basic Artisan Bread Recipe (BABR) on page 32, but includes these...

Ingredients:

2	tsp.	dried garlic granules (Do not use garlic powder or garlic salt.)
2	tsp.	fresh parsley leaves, washed, tougher stems removed and minced (You can substitute dried parsley leaves. Do not use dried parsley powder.)

From the BABR recipe, you need to remove this:

dash	whole seed mixtures for topping, like: raw caraway seeds, flaxseed, raw sunflower seeds, poppy and sesame seeds

Directions:

1. Follow BABR directions. But in step 2, incorporate the garlic granules and fresh parsley with the lukewarm water.

2. Proceed with the steps 3 to 14.

3. Skip step 15, then proceed with the remaining steps.

Garlicky Loaf

This recipe follows the Basic Artisan Bread Recipe (BABR) on page 32, but includes these...

Ingredients:

| 1 | tsp. | fresh garlic cloves, peeled, grated |
| 1 | tsp. | dried garlic granules (Do not use garlic powder or garlic salt.) |

From the BABR recipe, you need to remove this:

| dash | whole seed mixtures for topping, like: raw caraway seeds, flaxseed, raw sunflower seeds, poppy and sesame seeds |

Directions:

1.   Follow BABR directions. But in step 2, incorporate the fresh garlic and the garlic granules with the lukewarm water.

2.   Proceed with the steps 3 to 14.

3.   Skip step 15, then proceed with the remaining steps.

Raisin and Cashew Loaf

This recipe follows the Basic Artisan Bread Recipe (BABR) on page 32, but includes these...

Ingredients:

| 3 | tbsp. | raisins (You can substitute prunes, but make sure that the pits are removed. Mince the prunes.) |
| 2 | tsp. | raw cashew nuts, pounded or coarsely crushed |

From the BABR recipe, you need to remove this:

| dash | | whole seed mixtures for topping, like: raw caraway seeds, flaxseed, raw sunflower seeds, poppy and sesame seeds |

Directions:

1.   Follow BABR directions. But in step 2, incorporate the raisins and crushed cashew nuts with the lukewarm water.

2.   Proceed with the steps 3 to 14.

3.   Skip step 15, then proceed with the remaining steps.

Rosemary and Thyme Loaf

This recipe follows the Basic Artisan Bread Recipe (BABR) on page 32, but includes these...

Ingredients:

2	tsp.	fresh rosemary leaves, washed, dried, stems removed, and needles roughly minced (You can substitute 1 tsp. of dried rosemary. Do not use dried rosemary powder.)
2	tsp.	fresh thyme leaves, washed, dried, stems removed, and leaves roughly minced (You can substitute 1 tsp. of dried thyme. Do not use dried thyme powder.)

From the BABR recipe, you need to remove this:

dash	whole seed mixtures for topping, like: raw caraway seeds, flaxseed, raw sunflower seeds, poppy and sesame seeds

Directions:

1.   Follow BABR directions. But in step 2, incorporate the herbs with the lukewarm water.

2.   Proceed with the steps 3 to 14.

3.   Skip step 15, then proceed with the remaining steps.

Stove Top Flat Bread

You can very easily create your own flat bread without the need to bake these in the oven. Here is the basic recipe for stove top flat bread.

Follow the Basic Artisan Bread Recipe (BABR), but remove these:

| 2 | cups | cornmeal for dusting (plus a few more for dusting later) |
| | dash | whole seed mixtures for topping, like: raw caraway seeds, flaxseed, raw sunflower seeds, poppy and sesame seeds |

You would also need: rolling pin
thick bottomed skillet
spatula
knife
2 tea towels or thick-weaved paper towels
air tight container

Directions:

1. Follow BABR steps # 1 to # 5.

2. Skip step # 6.

3. Follow steps # 7 to # 8.

4. Once you have formed a ball, generously sprinkle a flat working surface with flour. Roll your dough into a thick log, then divide this into 8 equal sized disks.

5. With your hand cupped over the dough disks, roll these in a circular motion on the flat working surface until you have a relatively round ball of dough in your hand. Set aside.

6. Repeat step # 5 until you have rolled out 8 dough balls.

7. Dust flour on the rolling pin. Take one dough ball and roll it to a quarter inch thick disk. Make sure that you do not roll the dough too thinly. Add more flour if the dough sticks to the working surface or the rolling pin.

8. Repeat step # 7 until you have rolled out all the 8 dough balls.

9.   Heat the skillet on the stove top at the highest setting. Wait for it to become slightly smoky.

10.   Meanwhile, take an airtight container and line it with a tea towel. Reserve the other tea towel as "cover." If you are using paper towels, line the airtight container with one sheet. Every time a flat bread is cooked, line it with another paper towel.

11.   When the skillet is smoky, place one dough disk at the center of the heated surface. Cooking time should take no more than 1 minute on both sides. Flip the bread using a spatula. If and when the bread starts developing air pockets, simply press down on the dough with your spatula. The bread is done when you see patches of brown spots at the center of the flat bread. The edges should also be firm and not spongy.

12.   Remove the cooked flat bread from the skillet and place immediately on the towel lined container. Cover with the other tea towel. If you are using paper towels, you need another sheet to cover the cooked bread. This step actually helps cook the breads further without subjecting it to direct heat. Without this step, the flat bread becomes brittle and chewy.

13.   Repeat steps # 11 and # 12 until all the dough disks are cooked.

14.   Cover the last bread with the tea towel or paper towel and seal the container. Serve immediately or while the flat breads are still warm.

Soup and Stew Recipes

Asparagus, Corn, and Mushroom Soup

Ingredients:

1	pound	asparagus, washed, tough stalks trimmed, cut into 1½ inch long slivers
2	tbsp.	extra virgin olive oil
1½	cups	fresh corn kernels, washed and drained (You can substitute canned corn kernels but wash these thoroughly under running water to remove excess starch, salt and sugar. Drain well.)
1	piece	red bell pepper, medium-sized, washed, stem and seeds removed, minced
5	pieces	fresh *portobello* or button mushrooms, medium-sized, stalks removed, caps sliced into thin slivers
4	pieces	leeks, choose the white parts only, washed, roots removed, minced
2	cups	vegetable stock
½	tsp.	curry powder
-	-	salt to taste
-	-	ground pepper to taste
-	-	water, if needed

Directions:

1.   In a saucepan, heat oil until slightly smoky. Lower flame to medium setting. Stir-fry corn and bell pepper until pepper is limp, or about 3 minutes.

2.   Add in the leeks and mushrooms. Stir fry for another minute.

3.   Add the curry powder, vegetable stock and the asparagus. Season with salt and pepper. Add more water (half cup at a time) if you find the stock too heavy, too dense or salty. Allow the soup to boil for 10 minutes at the lowest flame setting, covered.

4.   Remove saucepan from flame. Let this stand for 2 minutes to allow the corn to cook through.

5.   Ladle soup into bowls and serve immediately.

Barley and Mushroom Stew

Ingredients:

1	cup	pearl barley, washed and drained well (you can substitute scotch barley, brown or wild rice, or buckwheat groats.)
8	cups	water
2	tbsp.	extra virgin olive oil
1	piece	onion, large-sized, peeled and sliced thinly
½	oz.	dried *porcini* mushrooms, washed then soaked in water for at least 12 hours. Discard soaking liquid. Squeeze dry, then soak for another 30 minutes in water just before using. (You can substitute dried *shitake* mushroms.)
2	tbsp.	tomato sauce
1	piece	carrot, large-sized, washed, peeled, diced
16	stalks	celery, large-sized, washed, roots trimmed, finely chopped
-	-	salt to taste
-	-	black pepper to taste
2	tbsp.	fresh parsley, washed, coarsely chopped, for garnish

You would also need: slow cooker
tight mesh strainer or cheese cloth

Directions:

1.   Set the slow cooker on the lowest setting. Pour in the barley and the water. Place the lid on.

2.   In a skillet, heat the oil and stir fry the onion slices until these are limp. This should take no more than 3 minutes. Set aside.

3.   Meanwhile, squeeze the mushrooms dry. Discard the stems and roughly chop the caps before setting aside. Take its soaking liquid and run it through the tight mesh container (or cheesecloth) to remove the impurities. Set the liquid aside but discard the impurities.

4.   Carefully incorporate the cooked onions (and its oil,) the chopped mushrooms, the soaking liquid, carrots, celery and tomato sauce into the pearl barley. Stir gently and place the lid back on. Cook the stew 8 hours.

5.   Season to taste before serving. Garnish with chopped parsley. 9

Black Bean Vegan Soup

Ingredients:

For the salsa:

2	tbsp.	fresh cilantro, washed, coarsely chopped
2	tbsp.	fresh lemon or lime juice, use as much as the pulp as possible
1	piece	jalapeño pepper, washed, stem and seeds removed, chopped
1	piece	ripe mango, washed, peeled, stone removed, flesh diced
1	piece	shallot, medium-sized, peeled, washed and minced
-	-	salt to taste
-	-	pepper to taste

For the soup:

2	tbsp.	extra virgin olive oil
2	pieces	onion, large-sized, peeled and minced
1	piece	carrot, medium-sized, washed, peeled and minced
1	piece	celery stalk, washed, roots trimmed, minced
4	pieces	garlic cloves, peeled and minced
½	tsp.	ground coriander powder
½	tsp.	ground cumin powder
3	cups	vegetable stock
½	cup	freshly squeezed orange juice, use as much of the pulp as possible
1	can 15 oz.	black beans, rinsed thoroughly under running water, drained well
-	-	salt to taste

For the garnish:

¼	tsp.	ground black pepper powder, as garnish
⅛	tsp.	dried red pepper flakes, as garnish

You would also need: food processor or blender

Directions:

1.   To make the salsa: combine all the ingredients in a large bowl. Adjust seasoning according to taste. Chill.

2.   To make the soup: heat oil in a large thick bottomed saucepan. Add the garlic, onion, celery and minced carrots all at once. Sauté until celery is limp and diced onions are transparent, or about 3 minutes.

4.   Except for the salt, add all the remaining soup ingredients into the saucepan and allow soup to boil uncovered at medium flame. After 5 minutes, remove saucepan from heat. Adjust the taste by seasoning it with salt.

5.   Transfer the contents of the saucepan into the food processor and blend well.

6.   To serve: ladle a small measure of soup into a bowl. Top with salsa and serve with bread.

Corny Nutty Chili Stew

Ingredients:

2	tbsp.	extra virgin olive oil
2	pieces	onion, medium sized, peeled, coarsely chopped
2	pieces	garlic cloves, peeled, coarsely chopped
2	pieces	celery stalks, washed, roots trimmed, coarsely chopped
1	piece	green bell pepper, washed, stem and seeds removed, coarsely chopped
1	cup	fresh or frozen corn kernels, washed and drained well
1	can 28 oz.	tomato juice
1	can 15 oz.	tomato sauce
1	cup	water
1	can 15 oz.	kidney beans, washed under running water, drained well
1	cup	raw cashew nuts, whole, washed and drained well
1	cup	dark raisins
½	tsp.	chili powder (add more for a spicier stew)
½	tsp.	Tabasco sauce (add more for a spicier stew)
1	tsp.	ground cumin powder
1	piece	bay leaf, whole
1	tbsp.	fresh oregano, washed, stems removed, coarsely chopped (You can substitute 1 tsp. dried oregano leaves. Do not use dried oregano powder.)
1	tbsp.	fresh basil, washed, stems removed, coarsely chopped (You can substitute 1 tsp. dried basil leaves. Do not use dried basil powder.)
-	-	salt to taste
-	-	black pepper to taste

Directions:

1.   Heat oil in a Dutch oven. Sauté garlic and onions until onions are limp, and the garlic is aromatic.

2.   Add the rest of the vegetables: bell pepper, celery, and tomatoes. Stir fry for 1 minute. Stir in the rest of the ingredients except the cashew nuts, raisins, and the seasonings (salt and pepper.) Set the flame on high heat and wait for the cooking liquid to boil. Afterwards, reduce the heat to the lowest setting. Cook the stew for another 15 minutes, covered.

3.   Remove the lid and stir in cashews and raisins. Add salt and pepper to taste. If you want a spicier stew, add more chili powder and/or Tabasco sauce. Cook for 20 minutes or until cashews are tender. Remove from flame.

4.   Just before serving, fish out the bay leaf. Serve immediately.

Minted Chickpea Curry

Ingredients:

For the stew:

2	cups	dried chickpeas, washed and drained well
6	cups	water
1	tsp.	dried chili powder
1	tsp.	turmeric powder
1	piece	russet potato, washed, peeled and diced (You can substitute sweet potato.)
2	pieces	tomatoes, washed and coarsely chopped
½	cup	coconut milk
-	-	salt to taste

For the garnish:

¼	cup	fresh cilantro leaves, washed and coarsely chopped
¼	cup	fresh mint leaves, washed and coarsely chopped
1	piece	fresh jalapeño pepper, washed, stem and seeds removed, minced

You would also need: slow cooker

Directions:

1.   Set the slow cooker on its lowest setting. Place the chickpeas in and pour in the water. Cook covered for 8 hours or until chickpeas are fork tender.

2.   Remove the lid and place in the rest of the stew ingredients. Stir gently. Season to taste. Place the cooker's setting to medium. Let the stew cook for another hour.

3.   Serve while warm. Ladle stew into soup bowls and garnish liberally with the chopped cilantro and mint leaves. Add the chopped jalapeño pepper for a spicier stew.

Ratatouille

Ingredients:

2	tbsp.	extra virgin olive oil
2	pieces	garlic cloves, peeled and minced
1	piece	onion, medium-sized, peeled, sliced into wedges
1	piece	eggplant, medium-sized, washed, stem removed, diced
1	piece	green bell pepper, small-sized, washed, stem and seeds removed, diced
10	pieces	snap beans, washed, dried, ends and strings removed, diced
2	pieces	tomatoes, large-sized, cut into half to remove seeds, diced
1	piece	zucchini, medium-sized, washed, dried, ends removed, diced
1	tbsp.	fresh oregano leaves, washed, stems removed, minced
1	tbsp.	fresh basil leaves, washed, stems removed, minced
2	tbsp.	red wine vinegar
1	can 15 oz.	tomato sauce
1	cup	vegetable stock
-	-	salt to taste
-	-	ground black pepper to taste

Directions:

1.   In a large Dutch oven, heat the oil over medium flame. Add the onions and stir fry until onion wedges are transparent.

2.   Add the garlic and cook for another minute or until the onions are limp. Add the rest of the vegetables, except the snap beans. Pour in the red wine vinegar and stir once. Place the lid on the Dutch oven and allow the vegetables to cook for 10 minutes over low flame.

3.   After 10 minutes, toss in the snap beans, tomato sauce and vegetable stock. Return heat to medium flame. Cook for another 2 minutes, uncovered.

4.   Season vegetable stew with basil, oregano, salt and pepper. Adjust to taste. Remove Dutch oven from flame. Serve stew immediately.

Simple Black Bean Stew

Ingredients:

2	cups	dried black beans, washed and drained well
6	cups	water
½	cup	light soy sauce
2	tbsp.	toasted sesame oil (You can substitute plain sesame oil.)
-	-	salt to taste
-	-	pepper to taste

You would also need: slow cooker

Directions:

Except for the salt and pepper, place everything in the slow cooker. Set to the lowest setting and cook covered for the next 8 hours. Just before serving, season with salt and pepper, if needed.

Spicy Green Bean Stew

Ingredients:

2	tbsp.	extra virgin olive oil
2	pieces	onions, large-sized, peeled and coarsely chopped
1	lb.	green beans, washed, dried, ends and strings removed, chopped into 2 inch slivers
1	can 28 oz.	whole tomatoes
2	pieces	zucchini, small-sized, washed, ends removed, chopped into 2 inch long slivers
1	piece	Hannah sweet potato, large-sized, washed, peeled and cubed (You can substitute: Japanese sweet potato or jewel yam. Russet potato can also be used in a pinch.)
¼	cup	water (or more, as needed)
-	-	dried cayenne pepper powder to taste
-	-	salt to taste
-	-	black pepper to taste
½	cup	flat leaf parsley, washed, stems removed, coarsely chopped, for garnish

Directions:

1.   In a thick bottomed skillet, heat oil over medium flame. Sauté the onion until it turns transparent. Carefully stir in the contents of the canned whole tomatoes. Gently break the whole tomatoes into smaller pieces using your cooking spoon.

2.   Add the sweet potato to the skillet. Pour in the water. Season to taste. Use more cayenne pepper powder if you want a spicier stew.

3.   Turn the heat up to the highest setting to let the stew boil. Once it starts to boil, put a lid on the skillet and then turn the flame down to the lowest setting. Let the sweet potatoes cook thoroughly. This should take between 35 to 45 minutes.

Note: After 15 minutes, check to see if there is still enough cooking liquid in the skillet. If the stew is becoming too dry, simply add more water ½ cup at a time. Pierce the sweet potato with a fork to see if it is done.

4.   When potatoes are cooked, add the zucchini and the green beans. Stir and allow to simmer for the next 7 to 10 minutes, covered. Check to see if the zucchini

can be pierced through after 7 minutes. If so, remove the stew from the heat immediately. If not, let it cook some more. Again, keep a careful eye on the cooking liquid. Add more water, but only if the stew is too dry. Season to taste again.

5.   To serve: ladle hot stew into individual bowls. Garnish generously with chopped parsley leaves, and pair this with freshly made flat bread.

Tofu in *Miso* Soup

Ingredients:

6	cups	vegetable stock
¼	cup	brown or red *miso* paste (You can easily buy this in the Asian section of your local grocery store. Do not use the instant or powdered *miso.*)
1	knob	ginger, thumb-sized, peeled and grated, stringy bits removed
20	pieces	snow peas, washed, ends and strings removed
4	pieces	fresh *shitake* mushrooms, large-sized, stems removed, caps sliced thinly (You can substitute dried *shitake* mushrooms but you need to soak these overnight before using.)
1	piece	carrot, medium-sized, washed, peeled, grated
2	pieces	green onions or leeks, washed, roots trimmed, minced
1	piece	red bell pepper, small-sized, washed, stem and seeds removed, minced
1	tsp.	sesame oil
-	dash	dried red pepper flakes
1	package 12.3 oz.	extra firm tofu, rinsed gently under running water, drained and sliced into ½ inch cubes
-	-	cilantro, washed, stems removed, minced, for garnish
-	-	salt to taste
-	-	white pepper powder to taste

Directions:

1.   In a small bowl, mix the *miso* paste with 1 cup of vegetable stock. Do this until you have a smooth but runny paste. Pour this, along with the rest of the vegetable stock and the grated ginger into a Dutch oven. Set this over high flame and bring to a boil.

2.   Add all the vegetables and mushrooms. Reduce heat to the lowest setting. Cover Dutch oven with a lid and cook for 20 minutes, or until carrots can be pierced with a fork.

3.   Stir in the red pepper flakes and the sesame oil. Season with salt and pepper.

4.   To serve. Place a few cubes of tofu into individual bowls. Ladle steaming hot *miso* soup on top and garnish with chopped cilantro. Serve immediately.

Juices, Smoothies and other Beverages

Banana-Strawberry Smoothie

Ingredients:

1	cup	water, add more if desired
½	cup	crushed ice, add more if desired
2	pieces	bananas, large-sized, peeled, flesh sliced in half
1	pound	strawberries, washed, stems removed (You can substitute other berries.)

You would also need: blender

Directions:

Blend everything until smooth. If the drink is too thick, add ¼ cup of water and blend once more. If it is too runny, add more ice. Serve immediately.

If you prefer a sweeter smoothie, simply add one or more bananas to the recipe.

Berry Elixir

Ingredients:

1	cup	water, add more if desired
½	cup	crushed ice, add more if desired
1	cup	fresh or frozen strawberries, washed, stems removed
1	cup	fresh or frozen blueberries, washed, stems removed
1	cup	fresh or frozen raspberries, washed, stems removed
1	piece	cucumber, washed, peeled, halved, seeds scooped out
1	piece	lemon, take as much of the zest as possible, seeds removed, squeeze as much juice and lemon as you can

You would also need: blender

Directions:

Blend everything until smooth. If the drink is too thick, add ¼ cup of water and blend once more. If it is too runny, add more ice. Serve immediately.

Berry Red Drink

Ingredients:

1	cup	crushed ice, add more if desired
½	cup	raspberries, washed, stems trimmed, halved
½	cup	strawberries, washed, stems trimmed, halved
½	cup	blackberries, washed, stems trimmed, halved
1	piece	apple, large-sized, washed, cored and cubed
1	piece	orange, peeled, membrane and seeds removed
½	piece	red beet root, washed, peeled and chopped
1	tbsp.	freshly squeezed lemon or lime juice

You would also need: blender

Directions: Blend everything until smooth. Serve immediately.

Berry Infusion

Ingredients:

½	cup	fresh blueberries, stems removed, washed, drained well
½	cup	fresh strawberries, stems removed, washed, drained well
½	cup	frozen blackberries, stems removed, washed, drained well
½	cup	frozen cranberries, stems removed, washed, drained well
1	cup	water
-	-	crushed ice
-	-	mint leaves, washed, stems removed, for garnish

You would also need: pitcher with lid or mason jar, thoroughly cleaned wooden spoon

Directions:

1.   Pour all the berries into the pitcher. Bruise these using a wooden spoon to help them release their flavor into the water.

2.   Pour the water in and mix well with the wooden spoon.

3.   Add enough crushed ice to fill the pitcher. Put the lid on, and let the berries' flavors infuse into the water for at least 3 hours.

4.   Serve with mint leaf garnish.

Blackberry Sage Water Infusion

Ingredients:

½	cup	fresh sage leaves, washed, squeeze dried
2	cups	fresh blackberries, washed, halved
2	cups	water
-	-	crushed ice
	sprig	sage leaf for garnish

You would also need: pitcher with lid or mason jar, thoroughly cleaned
wooden spoon

Directions:

1.   Place the raspberries into the pitcher. Mush these slightly using the wooden spoon.

2.   Place the sage into the pitcher. Bruise these using the wooden spoon.

3.   Add the water into the pitcher and stir well.

4.   Add enough crushed ice to fill the pitcher. Put the lid on, and let the flavors infuse into the water for at least 3 hours.

5.   Serve with sage leaf garnish.

Citrus Water

Ingredients:

½	piece	grapefruit, washed, quartered, visible seeds removed
1	piece	lemon, washed, quartered, visible seeds removed
1	piece	lime, washed, quartered, visible seeds removed
1	piece	orange, washed, quartered, visible seeds removed
1	cup	water
-	-	crushed ice
-	-	mint leaves, washed, stems removed, for garnish

You would also need: pitcher with lid or mason jar, thoroughly cleaned
wooden spoon

Directions:

1.   Squeeze the juices of the citrus fruits into the pitcher, then throw in the quartered slices. Try to fish out as much seeds as possible.

2.   Pour the water in and mix well with the wooden spoon.

3.   Add enough crushed ice to fill the pitcher. Put the lid on, and let the fruits' flavors infuse into the water for at least 3 hours.

5.   Serve with mint leaf garnish.

Cranberry Slush

Ingredients:

1	cup	water, add more if desired
½	cup	crushed ice, add more if desired
3	pieces	bananas, large-sized, peeled, flesh sliced in half
1	cup	fresh cranberries, washed, stems removed

You would also need: blender

Directions:

Blend everything until smooth. If the drink is too thick, add ¼ cup of water and blend once more. If it is too runny, add more ice. Serve immediately.

If the slush is too tart, either add more bananas to the recipe, or lessen the amount of cranberries.

Fruity Coconut Mix

Ingredients:

½	cup	crushed ice, add more if desired
2	cups	seedless grapes, washed, stems removed (You can use any variety of grapes as long as you carefully remove the seeds within.)
1	piece	apple, large-sized, washed, cored and coarsely chopped
1	piece	orange, medium-sized, washed, peeled, membrane and seeds removed, include juice
1	piece	young coconut, scrape the meat and juice

You would also need: blender

Directions:

Blend everything until smooth. Add more ice if the drink is too runny. Serve immediately.

Grapefruit Elixir

Ingredients:

1	cup	water, add more if desired
½	cup	crushed ice, add more if desired
1	cup	fresh grapefruit juice, seeds removed, squeeze as much juice and pulp as you can
1	cup	fresh or frozen berries of your choice, stems removed

You would also need: blender

Directions:

Blend everything until smooth. If the drink is too thick, add ¼ cup of water and blend once more. If it is too runny, add more ice. Serve immediately.

Mango Kale Smoothie

Ingredients:

1	cup	water, add more if desired
½	cup	crushed ice, add more if desired
4	pieces	fresh kale leaves, large-sized, washed, dried and torn
2	pieces	mangoes, large-sized, washed, stone removed, flesh scooped out

You would also need: blender or juicer

Directions:

Blend everything until smooth. If the drink is too thick, add ¼ cup of water and blend once more. If it is too runny, add more ice. Serve immediately.

Minty Pineapple Water

Ingredients:

2	cups	fresh pineapple chucks, cored, reserve as much as of its juice as possible
1	sprig	mint, washed, root and other woody bits trimmed off
1	cup	water
-	-	crushed ice

You would also need: pitcher with lid or mason jar, thoroughly cleaned wooden spoon

Directions:

1.   Place the pineapple chunks into the pitcher. Using a wooden spoon, try to break the chunks into smaller pieces without completely turning these into pulp.

2.   Add the mint sprig and bruise some of the leaves using the wooden spoon.

3.   Pour the water in and mix well.

4.   Add enough crushed ice to fill the pitcher. Put the lid on, and let the flavors infuse into the water for at least 3 hours.

Pear and Dates Drink

Ingredients:

1	cup	water, add more if desired
½	cup	crushed ice, add more if desired
2	pieces	pears, large-sized, washed, cored and cubed
2	pieces	soft dates, pitted
¼	head	fennel, washed, roots trimmed, coarsely chopped
¼	tsp.	vanilla extract

You would also need: blender

Directions:

Blend everything until smooth. If the drink is too thick, add ¼ cup of water and blend once more. If it is too runny, add more ice. Serve immediately.

Raspberry Lime Water Infusion

Ingredients:

2	pieces	fresh limes, washed, quartered
1	cup	fresh raspberries, washed, stems removed, halved
2	cups	water
-	-	crushed ice
	sprig	mint leaf for garnish

You would also need: pitcher with lid or mason jar, thoroughly cleaned
wooden spoon

Directions:

1.   Place the halved raspberries into the pitcher. Mush these slightly using the wooden spoon.

2.   Squeeze the limes into the pitcher, then throw in the spent lime quarters into the pitcher as well.

3.   Add the water into the pitcher and stir well.

4.   Add enough crushed ice to fill the pitcher. Put the lid on, and let the flavors infuse into the water for at least 3 hours.

5.   Serve with mint leaf garnish.

Spicy Blueberry and Banana Drink

Ingredients:

1	cup	water, add more if desired
½	cup	crushed ice, add more if desired
2	cups	fresh or frozen blueberries, washed, stems removed
2	pieces	bananas, large-sized, peeled, flesh sliced in half
¼	tsp.	ground cardamom powder
⅛	tsp.	ground cinnamon powder

You would also need: blender

Directions:

Blend everything until smooth. If the drink is too thick, add ¼ cup of water and blend once more. If it is too runny, add more ice. Serve immediately.

Spiked Apple Juice

Ingredients:

1	cup	water, add more if desired
½	cup	crushed ice, add more if desired
2	pieces	apples, large-sized, washed, cored and cubed
1	piece	carrot, large sized, washed, peeled and cubed
1	piece	celery stalk, medium-sized, washed, coarsely chopped
2	tbsp.	freshly squeezed lemon juice, use as much of the pulp as possible

You would also need: blender

Directions:

Blend everything until smooth. If the drink is too thick, add ¼ cup of water and blend once more. If it is too runny, add more ice. Serve immediately.

Spiked Green Tea Smoothie

Ingredients:

1	cup	water, add more if desired
½	cup	crushed ice, add more if desired
1	cup	green tea or *macha* powder
1	handful	baby spinach leaves, washed, dried and torn
1	piece	apple, medium-sized, washed, cored and cubed
2	pieces	bananas, medium-sized, peeled, flesh sliced in half
-	dash	nutmeg powder

You would also need: blender

Directions:

Blend everything until smooth. If the drink is too thick, add ¼ cup of water and blend once more. If it is too runny, add more ice. Serve immediately.

Vanilla Kiwi and Spinach Smoothie

Ingredients:

1	cup	water, add more if desired
½	cup	crushed ice, add more if desired
1	handful	fresh baby spinach, washed, dried and torn
5	pieces	kiwi, medium-sized, washed, and peeled
2	pieces	bananas, peeled, flesh sliced in half
½	tsp.	vanilla extract

You would also need: blender

Directions:

Blend everything until smooth. If the drink is too thick, add ¼ cup of water and blend once more. If it is too runny, add more ice. Serve immediately.

Watermelon Rosemary Water Infusion

Ingredients:

¼	cup	fresh rosemary leaves, washed, stems removed
½	piece	fresh watermelon, flesh scooped out, reserve as much of the liquid as possible
2	cups	water
-	-	crushed ice

You would also need: pitcher with lid or mason jar, thoroughly cleaned
wooden spoon

Directions:

1.   Place the scooped watermelon and juices into the pitcher.

2.   Place the rosemary leaves into the pitcher. Bruise these slightly by pounding the needles using the wooden spoon.

3.   Add the water into the pitcher and stir well.

4.   Add enough crushed ice to fill the pitcher. Put the lid on, and let the flavors infuse into the water for at least 3 hours.

5.   Serve with sage leaf garnish.

Veggie Burger Recipes

Black Bean and Potato Patties

Ingredients:

4	pieces	red or Russet potatoes, large-sized, skin left intact, sliced into large chunks, boiled until fork tender, cooled completely at room temperature or chilled (You can do this in advance.)
1	package 12.3 oz.	extra firm tofu, drained and pressed to remove excess liquid
1	can 15 oz.	black beans, washed thoroughly under running water, drained
¼	cup	peanut butter
4	stalks	scallions, washed, roots trimmed and minced
2	tbsp.	dried red pepper flakes
2	pieces	garlic cloves, peeled and minced
1	tsp.	green curry paste
1	tsp.	*Sriracha* sauce or any hot sauce you prefer
¼	tsp.	dried coriander powder
¼	cup	whole wheat pastry flour
-	-	salt to taste
-	-	pepper to taste

You would also need: oven
non-stick baking sheet/silicone mat on a regular baking sheet
fork or masher
aluminum foil
spatula

DIRECTIONS:

1.   Preheat your oven to 350°F or 175°C.

2.   Using your fingers, break the tofu into smaller chunks into a large bowl. Add the drained beans, curry paste, garlic, peanut butter, red pepper flakes, scallions, *Sriracha* sauce and coriander powder. Mix well. Season with salt and pepper.

3.   With a fork or masher, mash potatoes in a separate bowl. Then transfer the lot to the bowl with the black beans. Knead mixture until everything is well incorporated. Add the flour ¼ cup at a time. What you need is a mixture that is slightly wet and can

easily be formed into patties. If the mixture is too dry or has too much flour, it will crumble when you bake it. You do not have to use all the flour.

4.   Form 10 patties. Place these on the baking sheet and cover with aluminum foil. Bake one side for 15 minutes. Afterwards, remove the baking sheet from the oven, flip the burgers with a spatula and return to cook for another 15 minutes, covered. In the last 3 minutes of its baking time, carefully remove the foil to give the patties a brown outer layer. Let this rest for 2 minutes out of the oven before serving.

Masala **Burger**

Ingredients:

1	cup	fully cooked lentils
$^2/_3$	cup	water
2	tbsp.	olive oil
1	tsp.	*garam masala*
½	tsp.	cumin powder
-	-	salt to taste
-	-	pepper to taste
-	-	vegetable oil for frying

You would also need: skillet
                        paper towels

Directions:

1.   Mix all the ingredients together, except for the frying oil. Season well with salt and pepper. Form into 4 patties.

2.   Set the skillet over high flame. Wait for the oil to heat up a bit. Add enough vegetable oil to generously coat the bottom of the pan. Gently slide in the patties and fry for 5 minutes on the first side, and 3 minutes on the other. Transfer cooked patties onto paper towels to remove excess oil. Serve immediately.

Three Pepper Burger Patties

Ingredients:

2	tbsp.	vegetable oil
6	pieces	shallots, medium-sized, peeled and minced
6	pieces	canned *portobello* or button mushroom, large-sized, washed under running water, drained, minced
1	piece	green bell pepper, small-sized, stem and seeds removed, minced
1	piece	red bell pepper, small-sized, stem and seeds removed, minced
1	piece	yellow or orange bell pepper, small-sized, stem and seeds removed, minced
3	cups	cooked brown rice, cooled completely
2	tbsp.	peanut butter
3	tbsp.	sesame oil
1	tsp.	cumin powder
1	tbsp.	*Sriracha* sauce or any hot sauce you prefer
-	-	salt to taste
-	-	cornstarch (optional)

You would also need: wok
                                   oven
                                   baking sheet with nonstick surface or silicone mat
                                   saran wrap
                                   spatula

Directions:

1.   Over high flame, preheat the wok until it is slightly smoky. Stir fry the 3 bell peppers, mushrooms and onions for 3 minutes. Turn heat off.

2.   Toss the cooked rice, cumin powder, peanut butter, sesame oil and the *Sriracha* sauce into wok. Make sure that everything is well distributed. Allow this to cool completely at room temperature.

3.   Transfer the cooled pepper-mushroom mix to a glass bowl and cover with a saran wrap. Refrigerate this for at least 20 minutes before shaping the mixture into patties. It would be preferably though if this could be chilled overnight.

4.   When you are ready to bake, preheat oven to 350°F or 175°C. Spray cooking oil on a non-stick baking sheet, or on the silicone baking mat. (You can also use parchment paper on a cookie sheet.)

5.   Form the pepper-mushroom mixture into patties. If the patties are too wet, add a tablespoon of cornstarch at a time. Mix well. This batch should yield 8 burgers.

6.   Place burger patties onto the baking sheet and slide into the oven to cook for 15 to 20 minutes, uncovered. Using a spatula, flip the burgers and bake for another 15 minutes. Once cooked, remove baking sheet from the oven, and allow to cool slightly before serving.

Wheat Free Sweet Potato Burger

Ingredients:

6	pieces	sweet potatoes, large-sized, washed, peeled and julienned, soaked in cold water to prevent discoloration, drained well before using, squeeze out excess moisture using a tea towel
1	piece	onion, large-sized, peeled and minced
1	piece	green or red bell pepper, medium-sized, washed, stem and seeds removed, minced
1	piece	yellow or orange pimiento, small-sized, washed, stem and seeds removed, minced
3	cups	chickpea flour (You can also substitute cornmeal or oat flour.)
1	cup	cashew sour cream or any non-dairy sour cream substitute (You can substitute ordinary sour cream in a pinch.)
-	-	salt to taste
-	-	pepper to taste
-	-	vegetable oil for frying

You would also need: tea towel
paper towels

Directions:

1.   In a large mixing bowl, combine bell pepper, onions, pimiento, sour cream, with the drained sweet potatoes. Season well with salt and pepper.

2.   Incorporate the chickpea flour one cup at a time. Mix well with each addition. This should yield a very wet mixture. Adjust the taste as you go.

3.   Meanwhile, heat a skillet with enough cooking oil to generously coat the bottom of the cooking surface. On medium heat, allow the oil to become slightly smoky.

4.   With floured hands, scoop a handful of the sweet potato mix and form into patties. Drop patties in the heated oil and fry for 3 to 5 minutes. Cooking time would depend on how thick your patties are.

5.   Place cooked patties on absorbent paper towels to remove excess oil. You can serve this with your favorite vegetable salad and/or bread, with slices of fresh tomatoes and cucumber on the side.

Vegan Friendly Desserts

Apple Cake

Ingredients:

For the cake:

1½	cups	all purpose flour, sifted
2	tsp.	baking powder
½	tsp.	baking soda
1	cup	granulated sugar (You can substitute any baking-friendly artificial sweetener of your choice.)
½	cup	olive oil
½	cup	freshly squeezed apple juice, add the pulp if possible
2	tbsp.	maple syrup
2	tsp.	apple cider vinegar
1	tsp.	ground cinnamon powder
1	tsp.	zest of freshly grated orange
5	pieces	apples, medium-sized, washed, cored, diced
½	tsp.	ground nutmeg powder
½	cup	raw walnuts, coarsely chopped (optional)
¼	cup	dark raisins (optional)
-	-	oil for brushing
-	-	flour for dusting

You would also need: oven
9 inch spring form pan
wire whisk
wooden spoon
wire rack

Directions:

1.   Preheat the oven to 350°F or 175°C.

2.   Lightly oil the sides and bottom of the spring form pan. Lightly dust the oiled surfaces with flour. Set aside.

3.   In a large mixing bowl, sift the baking powder, baking soda and the flour together.

4.   In another bowl, combine the sugar and the olive oil and whisk until you have a smooth consistency. Whisk in the apple juice, cinnamon powder, maple syrup, vinegar and the orange zest. Add this to the flour mixture using a wooden spoon. Mix just enough to incorporate the wet ingredients with the dry.

5.   Fold in the apples and the nutmeg powder. Fold in also the raisins and walnuts if you are using these.

6.   Pour the cake batter into the prepared spring form pan. Tap the pans lightly on the kitchen counter to let out the air bubbles. Bake for an hour or until an inserted toothpick at the center of the cake comes out clean.

7.   Remove cake from oven, and place spring form pan on wire rack. After 30 minutes, remove the spring form pan, and set the cake on the wire rack to help it cool further. If possible, chill the cake before slicing and serving.

Banana Berry with Cashew Crisps

Ingredients:

2	cups	all purpose flour
1	tsp.	baking powder
½	tsp.	baking soda
½	tsp.	ground cinnamon powder
½	tsp.	kosher or sea salt
4	pieces	overripe bananas, large-sized, peeled, flesh mashed with a fork
¾	cup	brown sugar (You can substitute any baking-friendly artificial sweetener of your choice.)
$1/3$	cup	granulated sugar (You can substitute any baking-friendly artificial sweetener of your choice.)
½	cup	olive oil
¼	cup	unsalted cashew nut butter (You can substitute almond or *macadamia* nut butter.)
1	tbsp.	soy milk
1	tsp.	almond extract
¾	cup	raw cashews, coarsely chopped
$1/3$	cup	dried cranberries
-	-	oil for brushing

You would also need: oven
3 cookie sheets or silicone mat
wooden spoon
wire rack
wire whisk

Directions:

1.   Preheat the oven to 300°F or 175°C.

2.   Lightly brush 3 cookie sheets with oil. Set aside.

3.   In a large mixing bowl, combine baking powder, baking soda, cinnamon powder, flour and salt. Mix well with a wooden spoon. Make a well in the center of the flour mixture.

4.   In another bowl, whisk together the mashed bananas, the 2 types of sugar, olive oil, and nut butter. Try to incorporate as much air as possible to the mixture to give the cookies a lighter consistency. Whisk in the almond extract and the soy milk.

5.   Pour the liquid ingredients into the center of the flour mixture. Use the wooden spoon to mix everything. Fold in the cashews and the cranberries.

6.   Scoop a tablespoon of the dough and drop this on the oiled baking sheets. Leave enough spaces in between, about 3 inches apart. This would allow the cookies to spread out a little during the baking process.

7.   Bake in the hot oven for 10 to 15 minutes, or until the edges of the cookies turn golden brown. Remove baking sheets from the oven. Cool slightly. Using a spatula, scoop each cookie and place it on the wire rack to cool. Serve warm.

Carrot Spice Cake

Ingredients:

1¹/₃	cups	all purpose flour
1	tsp.	baking powder
½	tsp.	baking soda
½	tsp.	rock salt or kosher salt
1	cup	granulated sugar (You can substitute any baking-friendly artificial sweetener of your choice.)
½	cup	olive oil
¹/₃	cup	soy milk (You can substitute your choice of dairy-free milk.)
¼	cup	applesauce
2	tsp.	ground cinnamon powder
1	tsp.	vanilla extract
½	teaspoon	ground nutmeg powder
2	pieces	carrots, large-sized, washed, peeled and finely grated
1	cup	raw walnuts, coarsely chopped (optional)
-	-	oil for brushing
-	-	flour for dusting

You would also need: oven
9 inch spring form pan
wire whisk
wooden spoon
wire rack

Directions:

1.   Preheat the oven to 350°F or 175°C.

2.   Lightly oil the sides and bottom of the spring form pan. Lightly dust the oiled surfaces with flour. Set aside.

3.   In a large mixing bowl, sift the baking powder, baking soda and the flour together. Add the salt and mix with a wooden spoon.

4.   In another bowl, combine the sugar and ½ cup of olive oil. Beat with a wire whisk until foamy. Pour in the applesauce, cinnamon powder, nutmeg, soy milk and vanilla extract. Mix well.

5.   Make a well in the center of the flour mixture. Pour the liquid ingredients into the well. Mix with a wooden spoon until just combined. Do not over mix. Gently fold in the carrots and the walnuts if you are using these.

6.   Pour cake batter into the prepared spring form pan and bake for 50 minutes, or until toothpick inserted at the center of the cake comes out clean. Remove spring form pan from the oven.

Place this on a wire rack to cool completely at room temperature, about an hour. Remove cake from spring form pan and the place on the wire rack for another 15 minutes. Serve immediately.

Corn and Berry Muffins

Ingredients:

1¼	cup	all purpose flour
¾	cup	coarse cornmeal
1/3	cup	granulated sugar (You can substitute any baking-friendly artificial sweetener of your choice.)
2	tsp.	baking powder
½	tsp.	baking soda
¼	tsp.	rock or sea salt
1	cup	soy milk
1/3	cup	canola oil
1	tbsp	orange zest, freshly grated
1	cup	fresh or frozen blueberries, washed under running water, drained well (You can use other berries of your choice.)

You would also need: oven
12 cup muffin pan with paper liners
wooden spoon
wire rack

Directions:

2.   Preheat the oven to 400°F or 200°C.

2.   Line the muffin cups with paper liners.

3.   In a large mixing bowl, combine baking powder, baking soda, cornmeal, flour, salt and sugar. Mix well, then make a well in the center of the flour mixture.

4.   Pour the canola oil, orange zest and soy milk in the well. Stir with a wooden spoon. Very gently, fold in the berries.

5.   Spoon cake batter into the muffin cups. Fill the muffin cups only halfway up.

6.   Bake in the hot oven for 18 to 20 minutes, or until the surface of the muffins turn golden brown. Remove muffin pan from the oven. Carefully remove each muffin and place on the wire rack to cool completely at room temperature, or about 30 to 45 minutes.

Chocolate Pumpkin Muffins

Ingredients:

1	cup	all purpose flour, sifted
1	tsp.	baking powder
½	tsp.	baking soda
1	tsp.	ground cinnamon powder
1	can 16 oz.	pure pumpkin
1	cup	granulated sugar (You can substitute any baking-friendly artificial sweetener of your choice.)
½	cup	canola oil
$^1/_3$	cup	soy milk
¾	cup	nondairy chocolate chips
½	cup	chopped walnuts, optional

You would also need: oven
12 cup muffin pan with paper liners
wooden spoon
wire rack

Directions:

3.   Preheat the oven to 350°F or 175°C.

2.   Line the muffin cups with paper liners.

3.   In a large mixing bowl, sift together flour, baking powder, baking soda, and cinnamon powder. Make a well at the center.

4.   Add in the oil, pumpkin, soy milk and sugar. Mix well with a wooden spoon. Gently fold in the chocolate chips and the walnuts if you are using these.

5.   Spoon cake batter into the muffin cups. Fill muffin cups only halfway.

6.   Bake in the hot oven for 25 to 30 minutes, or until the surface of the muffins turn golden brown. Remove muffin pan from the oven. Carefully remove each muffin and place on the wire rack to cool completely at room temperature, or about 30 minutes.

Made in the USA
San Bernardino, CA
02 April 2017